FASTING WITH FERVOR

30 Days Toward a Lifelong IF Love Affair

WRITTEN BY SUSANNAH JUTEAU M.SC. RD
WITH KIM SMITH

An Unbelievable Freedom Book

Everyone tends to remember the past with greater fervor as the present gains greater importance.

ITALO SVEVO

Let's switch that to our present and our future having the greatest importance!

SUSANNAH

Table of Contents

Welcome from Kim

Greetings!

The 11th Unbelievable Freedom Habit Guide is another dealing with fasting as a practice. It's called *Fasting With Fervor* and was written by Susannah Juteau, R.D. M.Sc. Because of the freedom that fasting has brought to my life, I've included several titles focused on its simple, transformational power. I know what fasting can do to align body, mind, and spirit in a place of optimal health. Fully embracing and cultivating a faster's' mindset creates long term success, and quoting Ryan's recent Habit Guide, "Fasting Is the Foundation" of true health.

So this brings me to the author I've chosen. I first heard Susannah's voice when she was a guest on Gin Stephens' *Intermittent Fasting Stories* podcast. She impressed me with how she'd embraced fasting for her health and turned it into a "mom hack", revitalizing life with her young daughters. She's a registered dietician who has studied human nutrition at the Master's level. While I'm a big believer in trusting our own experience and intuition to nourish ourselves, it's great to learn from someone who understands the science of how our bodies use what we feed them.

Susannah blends both perspectives. She has textbook knowledge of nutrition, and she lives an intermittent lifestyle personally. In this book, she'll share with you how turning your IF life into a love affair can bring health, happiness, and freedom. It's what this series is all about!

Enjoy Your Life,
Kim

Susannah Juteau M.Sc. RD encourages you to consult your healthcare provider before making any health-related change. This guide cannot be used as a replacement for consultation with your healthcare provider and does not constitute medical advice.

Fasting with Fervor! ♥

Welcome to Fasting with Fervor! I'm Susannah, and I'm a registered dietitian who has used fasting to transform my own health.

Fervor means having an intense and passionate feeling.

I want you to feel that way for fasting - I do!

So each day there is a different piece of coaching to help you love your fasts. I want you to really take the program seriously and do the action tasks each day. It's only 30 days long so play **FULL OUT!!**

For our first day, I want you to reflect on the **GET TO** mentality.

Too often, we say we "have to."

❯ I have to drive the kids to school

❯ I have to make supper for everyone tonight

❯ I have to eat well

❯ **I have to fast**

Be honest with yourself. Do you feel like eating well and intermittent fasting is a burden and something you HAVE to do? The first step is awareness. Then you GET TO flip that script in your head into a 'GET TO.' There are people who are starving in our world, there are people who would love to have a healthy meal each day. We get to eat well. We get to choose to intermittent fast or not.

Action step

I'd like you to journal on this today.

❯ What are 20 things you have to do each day

❯ Change those items into a 'Get to' mentality

I get to fast!

Happy fasting,

Susannah

Love where you're headed

What is your vision for your health 5 years from now?

Take some time to think deeply on this one. **In 5 years, where do you want to be?**

Example questions to form your vision:

❯ What will your health look like?

❯ What will your ideal body look like?

❯ What kind of clothes will you wear?

❯ What will your meals and your fasting look like?

❯ How will you feel?

❯ What will your energy level be like?

❯ What activities will you be able to do?

❯ How will you impact your family?

Action step

Connect with your vision because I will be asking you about this on our first coaching call. want you to be laser-focused and be able to describe to me **exactly** what you want.

This is the tool you use when you're having a bad day. Your vision is what you should be thinking about when you're deciding whether or not to end your fast early. Your vision is what you should be connecting with when you're about to emotionally eat, your vision is what you should tap into when you just want to snack on the couch and start again tomorrow...

Go deep **now** so we have time to focus on other things on our call.

Here's an example of what your vision could look like:

In 5 years...

I am filled with so much joy that my friends and family are constantly gathering around me to feed off my energy. I have lost weight sure, but more than anything I have regained my confidence, rediscovered my inner-self and stopped hiding. I wear bright purple pants just because I want to! Plus, I easily find ones in my size and don't dread going to try them on in the shop. I am a regular at Zumba and the instructor actually knows me by name because I'm so committed. Food no longer fills me with dread. I enjoy my meals, I adore regular fasting every day, sweets don't have a pull on me the way they used to and I never miss a supper meal with my family. My knee and back pain has gone away and I no longer vegetate on the couch as soon as I get home from work. Come to think of it, even my work gives me more satisfaction now that my energy has skyrocketed! I feel joyful, fulfilled and like I'm actually living my purpose rather than burdened by the world around me. I'm even planning my first vacation in a long time. I'm going to Costa Rica and better believe I'll be wearing a bathing suit out in public!

Time to change your story!

Yesterday we connected with our vision for ourselves 5 years from now. Your vision is upbeat, fun, joyful, accomplished **AND totally possible**.

Do you see that your vision for yourself is 100% possible?

If not, you'll need to pay extra attention to the mindset messages in this 30-day program.

So, in order to get to your vision, I need you to get REAL with yourself.

Why hasn't your vision happened? What's been getting in the way? What are the obstacles? Why are you **stuck!?**

Action step

I want you to write down <u>at least</u> 10 reasons. Small or big.

We get to reflect on them and then we get to move past them. Because you won't be getting anywhere if you are stuck in the same old story. Same old cycle.

That's boring.

Your old story hasn't gotten you anywhere. Your old story won't get you anywhere.

It's time to change the story!

Susannah

Set your intentions and 💕 your ways of being

So much about health and weight loss is about setting intentions... And yet, this is something we (as a society) rarely talk about.

Do you set your intentions and ways of being every day? Do you make declarations for the day as soon as you wake up?

If you're just going about your days as you usually do and only think about your goals when you're eating, it will take a while to achieve success.

Being healthy is much more than counting calories, paying attention to what foods we eat or the time that we eat it. Being healthy starts with our thoughts.

For many, this concept takes a while to process. But, we have almost 30 days of action left to practice new ways of being and making new habits stick. **Play full out!**

Let's be **SUPER** committed to doing what we say we're going to do.

So, what does that look like?

We're going to create a new contract for you.

Action step

Choose 3 words of being that are important to you:

Examples: Free, joyful, open, connected, loving, powerful, committed, authentic, passionate, courageous, confident, giving, intimate, responsible, trusting, vulnerable, energetic etc.

Your contract: **I am a _____, _____, _____ woman!** Ex: I am a free, open, joyful woman!

Now, here is the best way to start your day:

1. Say your contract to yourself several times until you *really* feel it: I am a ____, ____, ____ woman!

2. Set a declaration for the day. Ex: Today I will be connected to my coworkers, eat foods that fuel my body and commit to going for a walk at lunchtime.

Think about these two things a few times during the day. Sometimes you'll achieve everything you set out for the day, sometimes you won't. Simply reflect on **why not** (do NOT beat yourself up about it. That doesn't achieve anything. This is to be **neutral** reflection).

Then, spend each day more intentional than the last :)

Susannah

Love the commitment

This is the life you have created! Embrace it and recognize how fortunate you are. **AND** you get to change what isn't working well.

Intermittent fasting is flexible, fluid, and freeing. That's why I love the name 'Fasting for Freedom.' There are so many ways to tweak your fasting so that it works well for you. And what's really great is that your fasting pattern can be altered based on what's happening that week.

But here's where you need to be cautious...it's easy to make exceptions every day and then all of a sudden, you're not fasting at all.

Is that you? Do you make exceptions if there's free food in the staff room, an impromptu Starbucks run with a coworker, finishing up your kids' plate so you don't waste the food, eating late at night because you're pooped from the day?

Do you find yourself constantly coming up with excuses to BREAK your fast early (or not fast at all) and then justify them as completely **valid** excuses?

Are you just *fooling yourself* that you want to get healthier when really, you're not ready to make any changes?

If this is you, it's really important to bring yourself back to your vision, your intentions and your contract.

WHAT do you want to achieve long-term?

Identifying the most common situations where you're jeopardizing your success is essential for figuring out the solutions.

If you continue self-sabotaging your success, there isn't a program in the world that will get you to where you want to go.

Action step

List 20 times you've made an excuse to not continue your fasting as you had planned. Are there any patterns? Do you remember your thoughts and feelings? Journal on your reflections.

Onwards and upwards!

Susannah

♥ your challenges

This is a follow-up from yesterday...

As much as we don't want to constantly make excuses for not being able to complete our fasts, challenges most certainly will come up.

The key is to determine if the challenge is **an excuse** or rather **a valid reason** to break the fast early/not fast that day. To help you, look at:

❯ How frequently is this happening? Is this self-sabotage? (or even sabotage from others)

❯ Am I dealing with the reason behind the reason? (there always is one!)

❯ Am I following through on my commitment to myself or giving up as soon as it gets hard?

❯ Am I living my contract throughout the day or just when convenient?

❯ Am I trying to do too much at once? (Look at your priorities; health should always be up near the top!)

❯ Am I expressing how I'm feeling instead of eating how I'm feeling?

❯ Am I lone-wolfing it? (i.e. not asking for support/help)

Action step

Think of yourself as taking your challenges out of your body, looking at them, massaging them and putting them right back in. Those same challenges are more often than not still there but when you recognize them, you can take action steps to change them.

For instance: when you recognize that you're always lone-wolfin' it through life and feeling stretched thin as a result, you can start reaching out for support more often. This can take on many different forms, such as, having an accountability partner, a coach, asking your husband to do the dishes every night, hiring a house cleaner, watching less TV, etc.

In the end though, let's learn to embrace and **LOVE our challenges**. It's the challenges that give us insight into **WHAT** we need to change.

Breakdown to breakthrough!!

Love,

Susannah

P.S. Action step is to reflect on the questions above. Journal on them. Which one jumps out at you the most? The more you take time to reflect now, the faster it is to identify what's going on in the moment in order to *skip the self-sabotage.*

Embrace that it will never be perfect

If I got a dollar every time someone told me they'll **try** again tomorrow, or start again on Monday, or "I'll **try** to do 'x'," I'd be rich!

Life is now.

Start "again" right now!

When a challenge comes up that you would maybe handle differently next time, embrace it and move on. Re-commit each and every single time something gets in the way. Have a breakdown and then recommit. Breakdown, recommit.

This will happen forever. It's human nature. Unexpected things come up all the time. We can recognize the challenges for what they are, be aware of them instead of making excuses, determine if there's something in life we can change so that it doesn't happen again and then **move on**. That's the beauty of intermittent fasting, it's so flexible and there is no such thing as doing it "wrong" because everyone follows something a little different.

So, here's where this mentality of "failing" and "trying again" really comes from. **Perfectionism.**

This took me a while to get a handle on because I'm not a type A personality at all. I never cared if my essays were completely perfect before turning them in. I was always happy with "good enough" or "done is better than perfect." But when it comes to our food intake (or lack thereof in the case of fasting) and exercise, we've developed this notion of "good" and "bad."

I've been good today (Yay, gold star! ★).

Oh, I had a really bad week with food (I'm completely failing at this, I might as well quit now).

And we've learned to get down on ourselves when our food day hasn't gone perfectly.

THAT IS PERFECTIONISM!!

This is often what leads people to get overweight or unhealthy in the first place. Once we all realize that **no one eats perfectly** then we can all move on and be better for it.

And right now you're probably still thinking there are people who eat perfectly, right!?

I've been a dietitian since 2010, I've been in Neuroscience or Nutrition since 2001, I am surrounded by very healthy and fit people. <u>I have yet to meet a single person who eats perfectly</u>. Even those who think they do, just don't know what they don't know.

Food is amazing, food is nourishing, food is comfort, food is connection, food is health. But food does not need to be perfect to be all those things.

Action step

Reflect/journal on whether you let perfectionism get in the way of your success? Is this just another form of self-sabotage?

Accept yourself just as you are and let go of perfectionism.

● Susannah

♥ the ☼ and your mood

For the vast majority of people, our moods are directly correlated to the type of food we choose to eat and the quantity we eat.

Tomorrow I'll go over how fasting improves mood but I want to make today's <u>action step</u> really easy so you can catch up on the tasks from this past week.

I want you to take a walk outside. It doesn't matter if it's actually sunny out. The benefit of being exposed to natural light on our moods is huge.

As you walk, focus on all of the sounds around you. Focus on the sound of your feet hitting the pavement. Pay attention to whether there are birds chirping or not. Notice where your body feels tense and where it feels limber.

When was the last time you took a walk and noticed all of those things?

Possibly never?

If you're lucky enough to have a sunny day, connect with the feeling of calmness of serotonin being released. Serotonin is a hormone in the brain that is associated with boosting mood and helping people feel at peace and focused. When these serotonin levels dip, you're more at risk of seasonal affective disorder (SAD).

Additional sunlight benefits to think about:

❯ Stress fighting

❯ Builds strong bones

❯ Cancer prevention (moderate exposure to sun that is)

❯ Heals skin conditions

❯ Preliminary research shows links between sunlight and rheumatoid arthritis, lupus, IBS and thyroiditis

Enjoy your walks! ●

Susannah

P.S. I noticed in Grad school that I have SAD. Nowadays I am very conscious of how much sun light I'm getting in the winter months and if it's raining a lot, I use a Happy Light that works wonders!

Love IFs effect on mood

On those days where fasting feels particularly hard or you're tempted to end your window early it's great to connect with all of the reasons fasting is beneficial for your health.

The next series of messages will help you get there.

How fasting improves our mood:

❯ Fasting encourages the gut to release more serotonin. Serotonin is the feel-good hormone in our brain.

❯ There is an increase in GABA which is a calming neurotransmitter

❯ Fasting re-sensitizes dopamine (our "reward" hormone)

If you're not experiencing this boost in mood, there are likely a few reasons. Have you been fasting regularly for a month or more? Are you consistent with your fasting? How is the quality of food in your diet? Pairing WHAT we eat and WHEN are both essential for your health so make sure you're doing a combination in order to get results.

There is one other reason you may not experience a boost in mood. It's possible your body has become dopamine resistant (just like our bodies can become insulin resistant). If you're always on the go and consuming instantly gratifying activities such as social media notifications, sugar, binge-watching videos, always trying to learn new things etc. Then you're constantly stimulated day in and day out. You need a dopamine fast. Luckily it only takes 24-hrs to reset dopamine receptors.

To reset dopamine: Boredom is key. Put your phone down, stop watching TV, fast from food.

If this is raising some immediate excuses for why you can't do this, you need a dopamine fast more than anyone!

Action step

Reflect on whether or not you've experienced a boost in mood and determine why/why not.

Focus on how fasting can spread more joy in your life and to those around you and you'll be connected to the bigger purpose.

It's not just about you!

Fasting = Improved mood

XO,

Susannah

Love your gut

When our gut is out of whack, our mood is affected, our well-being is affected and our weight is affected!

It's extremely hard to lose weight (easy to gain though) when your microbiome is out of balance

Fasting is one of the best ways to readjust this balance.

When someone asks you why you're fasting, this is an excellent answer: "For my gut health." The majority of gut specialists now recommend intermittent fasting as the most EFFECTIVE way to change our microbiome! Here's why:

- There is a species of gut bacteria that thrives when we cut calories or don't eat anything

- Fasting increases gastro-intestinal microbiome diversity ("skinny" people have a much more diverse microbiome than those who struggle with their weight)

- Giving your gut a break from constantly digesting food allows for repair and cell clean up to happen

The other part of improving your gut health is to eat whole, nourishing foods that help the gut bacteria flourish.

Are you doing this?

Action step

Journal and reflect on how your food intake contributes to your gut or hinders it.

Questions to ask yourself: How often am I feeding my gut bacteria sugar? *Which bacteria will multiply when I do this?* How often am I feeding my gut processed food? Am I eating pre- and probiotics daily? How many fruits and vegetables am I eating a day? *should be 7+* Do I have a source of **fiber** every time I eat? How often do I make excuses for my intake? *Once in a while no big deal, if you're doing it regularly, you really need to tap into your vision again. Is health a priority in your life right now?*

Fasting = gut health

Stay consistent,

Susannah

Love your cells 🧬

The two biggest reasons to practice intermittent fasting are for the benefits that come from ketosis and autophagy.

Ketosis: The body enters ketosis when insulin and blood glucose levels are low enough to increase fat oxidation 🔥. Fat oxidation (burning fat) = increased ketone production. The longer we fast, the more the ketone levels can increase.

Autophagy: The process of cell clean up, waste removal, getting rid of damaged cells, cell repair and removal of toxins.

When we're thinking of the powerful effects of fasting on our cells, staying consistent becomes easier.

Fasting is so much more important than just losing weight.

Fasting helps our heart, our blood pressure, our insulin levels, our lipids, how long we live, our skin, our neurons, our mood, our energy, our focus, our gut, our metabolism, our immune system etc.

❯ I can come up with 50+ reasons to fast, the vast majority of which are backed up by science.

Get in tune with these benefits and focus on THEM. Focusing on how intermittent fasting will help you lose weight isn't very motivating...

Action step

Do a 15 minute meditation thanking your body and your cells for everything you do. And before you say you don't have time for a 15 minute meditation, think about that dopamine reset from yesterday's email... Slow down and MAKE TIME for this. Start with thinking about your brain cells, take deep breaths, count those breaths for a bit, settle into the gratitude practice of loving your body and go through each muscle group and organ. Don't forget the liver (size of a football!) which is responsible for filtering the blood and clearing all the toxins from your body.

Fasting = cell clean up

Susannah

♥ the alertness

How many of you think that by not eating you'll hit a point where you:

❯ Feel lethargic

❯ Won't be productive

❯ Won't have the energy to do exercise

❯ Have poor memory to perform at work

Now think of the last time you had a big meal. As in a meal where there was tons of delicious food and you wanted to try everything and ended up feeling quite stuffed.

Thanksgiving? Christmas?

How did you feel after that meal?

Likely all of the points above.

We've been led to believe that if we don't constantly eat we won't have the energy to perform day-to-day activities.

In all actuality, when we don't eat we become more alert! It all makes sense when you think back to our ancestors. If they didn't have food they had to be extra alert in order to find food and survive.

Here are the areas studies have shown food deprivation or intermittent fasting are beneficial for (around alertness that is, otherwise the list would go on forever):

❯ Sustained attention

❯ Additional ability to focus

❯ Improved simple reaction time

❯ Improved short-term memory recall

❯ Overall cognitive performance

❯ Ability to fall asleep

❯ Mood consistency

Action Step

Read those points above carefully and think about how they apply or could apply in your life. Too often we read facts, say "that's cool" and don't give any more reflection. We won't change or have new ways of being without deep reflection about what's working and what isn't so I invite you to go deeper.

Fasting = Increased Alertness

Happy Fasting,

Susannah

Love your muscles

Too often, I hear from people that they're not making time to do exercise on a DAILY basis. The struggle is real - for me as well. I absolutely love doing exercise and yet there are many days that time gets away from me.

I can't imagine how it would be if I didn't like exercise.

But here's the thing. If you want fasting to be extra beneficial for burning fat, then pairing exercise and fasting is a beautiful thing.

✦ ⚡■ Doing exercise causes our muscles to use up muscle glycogen. In order to refuel our muscle then takes glucose from the bloodstream allowing us to reach ketosis faster ⚡■✦

Action step

How can you incorporate more exercise in your day? If this makes you shudder and roll your eyes, then think of all the times you could be doing extra movement each day - parking further, going for a quick 5 min walk outside when you wake up, dancing as you make supper, stretching as you watch TV, shaking your legs as you read through emails, walking while you're on the phone. Make a list of 10 ways to incorporate movement in your day.

If exercise is easy for you, then ask yourself how you can uplevel your game. Are you doing something **EVERY** day? Are you challenging yourself to the next level? Something like signing up for a running race, is as much for your mental endurance as your physical. Having discipline in athletics easily applies to other areas → especially when you allow your mind to draw those parallels.

Exercising = Reaching ketosis sooner

Happy Fasting!

Susannah

Love the sleep 🌙

I often hear that people can't sleep on an empty stomach.

I'm pretty sure that's just the story they tell themselves...

Which then becomes true because they make it true.

Just like before I started intermittent fasting I told myself that I couldn't possibly skip breakfast and still function during the day, needed numerous snacks a day to avoid being hangry AND that I absolutely had to eat after a workout otherwise I'd feel faint!

All stories.

Truth is. Once we get past the mindset that we **can't** do something, that's where we get to experience a breakthrough.

Here's what some research shows:

❯ Food intake after dark = worsened sleep quality

❯ Adults who don't sleep well tend to have irregular eating behaviors such as more frequent, smaller, energy-dense and highly palatable snacks at night

❯ The more you match your eating to the biologic clock (sunlight), the better

❯ Shorter sleep duration = excess weight

Action step

Reflect - Has fasting improved your sleep? If not, what have you let get in the way? How much sleep are you allowing yourself to get a night?

Your weight and your health have to do with your **WHOLE** lifestyle, not just what you're eating and at what time. When I work with people in my year-long Mastermind, we work on every aspect of lifestyle and it's often something unexpected that's holding women back from achieving true freedom.

Fasting = Improved sleep

Happy Fasting,

Susannah

Live longer AND stay healthy!?

I want you to think of yourself at 80 years old.

Perhaps one of your parents is approaching that age right now?

Maybe one of your grandparents lived until 80?

How do you want to look when you're 80? More importantly, how do you want to FEEL?

Connect with your future self and all that you want to become. Imagine yourself without any age-related diseases. Imagine the only pills you're taking are vitamins - and because you want to, not because you need to.

How does Intermittent Fasting prolong your life-span and your health-span?

❯ Through increased autophagy (destruction or repair of damaged cells)

❯ Increasing mitochondrial efficiency

❯ Improved circulation

❯ Cardiovascular disease protection

❯ Improved brain function

Action step

It might sound silly but step into the future and pretend you are now 80 years old. Write a letter to your present self. Psychologically, this is one of the best ways to connect with your future and helps send home the idea that what you're doing right now with your health, deeply affect your future self.

Here's what that letter could look like:

Dear Susannah,

Believe it or not, I'm one of the most nimble old ladies in my group of friends. And most of them are 10 to 20 years younger than me! I'm so glad I smartened up in my 20s and focused on the food I was putting in my body instead of satisfying every craving that popped into my mind. My bloodwork comes back clear every year (I'm pretty sure I'm even healthier than my doctor), I have no ailments and I continue to practice intermittent fasting. It'll probably be shocking to you but I never needed surgery for that dang brain tumor again... I'm convinced fasting is what kept things from growing. I continue to be off headache meds too. I still need to fast regularly but after almost 50 years of it, it's really a no-brainer. In fact, I would likely feel quite sick if I had to eat all the time

Thank you for putting my health first so many years ago. As a result, I have passed on healthy eating habits to my girls (who have fully grown kids of their own now!) I still go for a walk every day and though my knees crack when I bend down, I can play on the floor when my great-grand children visit. I actually can't think of a single person I know who can still do that at 80! I feel joyful, free and more than anything... fulfilled.

XOXO

Don't forget about me!

Fasting = Longevity

Happy fasting,

Susannah

DAY 16

Love accountability

Are you a lone wolf?

When you have a stressful day, do you reach for food to feel better?

Or do you reach out? Focus out? Call a friend? Call a buddy?

One of the best reasons to work with a dietitian or a health coach over a long period of time is to have that person to reach out to when going through stress, frustration or overwhelm.

We all have breakdowns *every* day. But when we retrain our brains to reach out instead of reach inward, then those breakdowns can become breakthroughs.

Action step

Reach out to someone today. Ask them *what they're hoping to create with their health in the next year.* Don't be afraid to reach out to someone who doesn't look like you too. We are ALL seeking health goals.

I challenge you to just have that conversation with someone today. 👇■👇■

From there, maybe they'd be a great fit to be an accountability buddy! If not, try again tomorrow.

Success is achieved by reaching out and not trying to do everything on your own.

It also happens one step at a time - so be patient!

XO,

Susannah

Love Mindfulness

Mindfulness can be applied to many goals.

Mindfulness in your relationship, mindfulness and awareness of your surroundings, mindfulness of your feelings and your stress level, mindfulness of nature, etc.

Eating mindfully is an important aspect of health.

Michelle May, MD wrote an amazing book on mindful eating and here are the steps:

1. **Ask yourself why:** Am I physically hungry? Am I having cravings for a particular texture? Am I moody and looking for comfort? Am I feeling overwhelmed? Am I feeling pressured?

2. **Set an intention:** How will this meal or treat change my current status? How full do I want to feel? Do I want to feel differently mentally or emotionally?

3. **What do you need?:** What foods are available - what do I want and what do I need? Is it food that I seek for my current needs? If so, how much will I need to eat?

4. **Focused eating:** Reduce all possible distractions (TV, phone, computer, podcasts). Experience every bite. Take your time. Put your fork down in between bites. Pay attention to fullness cues.

5. **Check in:** Halfway through your meal, check in. Evaluate your physical, emotional and mental sensations. Did you reach the intention you set? If so, decide whether (and why) you wish to continue or, alternatively, stop eating. Do you have 'diet' voices telling you you've had enough when really you're still hungry? Or diet voices telling you that you can't eat this again tomorrow/again, so you better eat all of it. Are you feeling social pressure to keep eating? Perhaps you're loving the food so much that you want to keep eating?

Action Step

Ask these questions to yourself at each meal today/this week.

Mindful eating is all about reflection without judgement

If you have an eating experience that you don't want to repeat, you have the **POWER** to change it.

Instead of focusing on **BEING** good, focus on **FEELING** good.

These principles tie in so perfectly with intermittent fasting, don't they!?

FASTING = MINDFULNESS

Happy fasting,

Susannah

Love your food!

This next series of messages will be focused on nutrition and meals. WHAT you eat is just as important as WHEN you eat!

Food is delicious. Food is energizing. Food is social. Food is comforting. Food is nutritious. Food is fuel.

Food is an excellent addition to our lives and we should be enjoying it.

Food should be an addition to our lives, not a takeaway.

What I mean by that is we should love our food and love our meals rather than hate what we're eating or feel guilty because we ate a certain way.

Do you love your meals?

What do your meals look like when you're loving your meals? How do you feel? What about when you're hating them?

Action step

Journal on the above questions.

Here's an example to get you started.

When I'm loving my meals, I am eating together with my family. I have planned my meal ahead of time so I have all of the ingredients, I've let my girls help me with the prep and we all get excited to eat! I light the fireplace for some ambiance and possibly even put on some soft music. The meal is balanced with many colours of the rainbow on the plate. I know the food is not only nutritious but also delicious. I eat slowly and enjoy every bite. I have a glass of wine and I look forward to dessert! We all talk about our day and enjoy our time together. I feel satisfied, fulfilled, healthy, energized, joyful, comforted, safe.

When I'm hating my meals, I'm eating on the go. I grabbed a few snacks as I rushed out of the house and I have 10 minutes to eat while I drive. No one is with me. I don't particularly like anything and I definitely don't get any satisfaction from it. Before I know it, each item of food is finished and I don't even remember chewing. I still feel like I'm missing something - I seek a crunchy texture. Mmm chips! Or something sweet could work too actually... I haven't had a brownie in a while. I do have cookies at home though! That'll do for now. Overall I feel frustrated, rushed, dissatisfied, like a failure, bored, unfulfilled, like I'm missing something, lack of energy.

Now reflect.

What percentage of the time are you loving your meals in a week/month? What percentage of time are you ho-hum about your meals?

Now, what can you do about it?

XO,

Susannah

Love Balance ⚖️

Eating balanced meals can bring about so much freedom.

Freedom because, once you're paying attention to balance, nutrition just comes along for the ride and becomes easy rather than yet-another task to keep track of.

Action step

For your meals this week I want you to think of these questions. We'll dive into each one in the next few days.

1. Does your meal have a colourful balance?

2. Where are your sources of fiber?

3. Do you have a source of protein?

4. Are you including two different vegetables?

Think of this as an audit of your meals and then reflect on what can be done differently! Does that task feel heavy? Connect to your vision. Connect to your future-self one year from now. Is your health one of your top priorities right now? Nutritious meals play an integral part!

Balanced meals = Freedom

Susannah

Love all of the beautiful colors! 🌈

The easiest way to have a balance of micronutrient intake without having to count and keep track is to eat all colours of the rainbow each day.

Red Foods

❯ Benefits: Supports the urinary tract, DNA and protects against cancer and heart disease

❯ Phytonutrients: lycopene, ellagic acid, quercetin, hesperidin, anthocyanidins

❯ Examples: watermelon, tomatoes, grapefruit, pomegranate, raspberries etc

Purple/Blue Foods

❯ Benefits: Supports the heart, brain, bone and arteries. Fights cancer and allows for healthy aging

❯ Phytonutrients: resveratrol, anthocyanidins, phenolics, flavonoids

❯ Examples: plum, eggplant, dark grapes, blueberries, blackberries, red onion

Green Foods

❯ Benefits: Supports eye health, arterial function, lung health and liver function.

❯ Phytonutrients: lutein/zeaxanthin, isoflavones, EGCG, indoles, isothiocyanates, sulforaphane

❯ Examples: kale, broccoli, spinach, kiwi, avocado

White Foods

❯ Benefits: Supports healthy bones, circulatory system and arterial function

❯ Phytonutrients: EGCG, allicin, quercetin, indoles, glucosinolates

❯ Examples: onion, mushrooms, garlic, cauliflower

Yellow/Orange Foods

❯ Benefits: Supports eye health, immune function, gums, healthy growth and development

❯ Phytonutrients: alpha-carotene, beta-carotene, beta cryptoxanthin, lutein/zeaxanthin, hesperidin

❯ Examples: Squash, carrots, sweet potato, papaya, pineapple

Action step

Eat a *minimum* of one food from each colour group daily. A great way to do this is to aim for half of your plate to be vegetables at each meal!

XO,

Susannah

Your blood sugar loves you

During a fast, since you are not eating, it's only natural that blood sugar levels drop. As a result insulin levels drop which then improves your insulin sensitivity.

This is important because when glucose is in our bloodstream, we want insulin to be super effective at getting the glucose out of the blood and into the cells.

In today's society, we are constantly snacking/munching/grazing and as a result our insulin never has a break.

But as fasters, your body gets a break and your beta cells (which produce insulin) get a break.

So, your body thanks you every time you fast!

The next step is to get your body to thank you every time you eat as well.

The best way to do this is to pay attention to balance such as in the last emails but ALSO to notice when something you eat will spike your blood sugar.

Foods that spike blood sugar:

❯ Sweets

❯ Refined carbohydrates - bread, croissants, muffins, chips, rice etc

❯ Sugars - including the natural ones such as honey and maple syrup

❯ Most drinks - including juices

It's not necessary to put these foods completely off-limits. But you want to eat them **consciously, with intention** and **combine them with other foods** so that your blood sugar doesn't spike. Protein, fat and fibre all slow down the digestion of refined or processed foods.

Let's get deeper into protein, fat and fibre tomorrow.

Action step

Never eat refined/processed food on its own. Always include a source of protein, fat or fiber.

And for every food that you put in your body, ask: **Is it worthy!?**

Susannah 💕

Love all foods

I can virtually guarantee that everyone reading this has lived in the 80s.

So we all lived through many years of being told that fat is awful for our bodies, extremely high in calories, and to be avoided at all costs.

Most of us are still fearful of fat.

Fat does have more calories per gram than protein or carbohydrate but that doesn't mean we should be avoiding it.

Fat helps us absorb nutrients. Vitamins A, D, E and K can't be absorbed without fat.

Fat slows down digestion. So instead of foods being digested quickly and being absorbed right into the bloodstream - likely to cause a spike in blood sugar - the food takes its time to leave the stomach and be absorbed. Think of it as going from a sprint down to a peaceful stroll...

Protein and fiber also slow down digestion. The best meal is one that incorporates all three: Fat, protein and fiber. Adding some starchy vegetables or whole grains adds satisfaction and more nutrients as well.

Action step

My message for today is to be conscious when you label foods as good or bad. Where is that labelling coming from? Is it actually true? Does it serve you to think of foods that way?

It's time to be super conscious of your thoughts and to challenge them! It wasn't long ago that each of us believed we should be eating breakfast within an hour of waking up whether we were hungry or not... right?

Don't fear the fat.

Happy eating,

Susannah

Love the freedom

While on the topic of loving all foods...

I'm going to jump right into the action step!

Action step

1. Make a list of all the foods that cause guilt, shame, worry etc.

2. Explore the reasons you feel negatively about those foods

3. Eat a couple of the ones you feel particularly charged against

4. Challenge the thoughts and beliefs.

I don't believe in any food restrictions. Fasting is all about freedom! Freedom from food guilt. Freedom from labelling. Freedom from calories. Freedom from thinking you don't have all of the information you need.

I can't think of a single food I won't eat. There are many I don't particularly like and prefer not to eat like hotdogs and flavoured yogurt but I don't feel negatively towards those foods. I certainly don't feel I need to restrict them for any reason.

So often clients ask me "can I have this?" "oh, I better not eat that... right?" "You're going to judge me if I tell you what I ate."

I don't believe any food is off-limits.

Otherwise, there's the restriction mindset → *"but I really want it"* → "ok so I ate it but now I feel guilty" → "might as well keep "being bad" for the rest of the day!" → I'll start again on Monday...

Um, can you think of any of those thoughts that actually *serve* you? Help you achieve your goals? So what is the purpose of them? Ironically, the purpose is often **to justify to yourself that you <u>can't</u> do it.** Our brains do funny things to stay safe. We LOVE to stay comfortable. Stay in the status quo. Not have to make any real behaviour changes. *"See, my body can't lose weight."* *"I'm just addicted to sugar"* *"I'm just really bad at this."*

It's time to catch what you're saying to yourself and instead flip the script on its head. I damn-well **CAN** make changes and I **WILL**. You watch me.

I am a powerful, driven, free woman and I WILL succeed.

Yes, you are. And yes, you will.

XO,

Susannah

Love breaking the fast!

How excited do you get when you're about to break your fast!?

Like, super excited right!?

That meal after a fast is just so satisfying. The longer the fast, the more satisfying that meal is I find.

Do you make sure your 'breaking-fast' meal has been planned ahead so that you get to enjoy it even more than a regular meal?

Do you make sure it's a balanced meal and something you're looking forward to having throughout the day? Do you make it a little extra special with some nice napkins, or a candle, or some calm music? Maybe even look forward to a dessert to be included with the meal?

One of the best ways to improve your health AND enjoy your fasts is to plan your meals ahead of time.

Doing so ensures you are getting maximum nutrition from your meals and not overcompensating with food due to having fasted all day.

This is important whether you're fasting for 12 hours a day or for 5 days at a time.

Otherwise it's so easy to break a fast with snacks, grazing, overeating, seeking out certain food textures and overall feeling lost and unsatisfied.

Action step

Plan your 'breaking fast' meals each day this week. The weeks' planning can be done all at once or one day at a time. It can even be done the morning of. Don't let this make you feel overwhelmed - just do it and make it easy. It can be a scribble on a notepad even. The key is to plan ahead of time!

Meal Planning = Avoiding a less healthful "drive-through" dinner

Happy fasting. Happy eating.

Susannah

Embrace the emptiness

So many people report to me that they LOVE the feeling of stomach emptiness during a fast.

Sound like it's not coming from an obsessive/unhealthy standpoint either.

Many express the love of emptiness so it can be filled with Spirituality and focus on prayer, others express love of the feeling because they are more in tune with other feelings in their body, others love the breakf from constantly eating (and feeling food controls them rather than the other way around) and others still, love it because they are connected to fasting being beneficial to their health and that emptiness feeling acts as a reminder.

Do you also embrace the feelings of fasting?

Do you feel you embrace the clean fasts in order to get to this point, the extra time you have where you're not preparing meals and most importantly, all of the benefits that we discussed early on in this series?

In order to get to the point where we are **fasting with fervor** and truly loving intermittent fasting, it's ok to love the feeling of emptiness too.

Action step

I'd like you to journal on all of the things you love about being in a fasted state. How do you feel before you hit ketosis, how do you feel afterwards (usually around hours 14-16 of a fast, largely depending on your diet while eating)? Fasting doesn't always feel easy. In fact, contrary to what you hear on social media - many people hate the fasting but LOVE the feeling after the fast. So what feelings can you focus on during a fast that you do love?

Fast with Fervor!!

Happy fasting,

Susannah

Unconditional Love

I highly recommend you throw out the scale.

Or hide it under your bed at least.

Women often tell me they weigh themselves every day so they can catch themselves the moment they gain weight. I call BS.

The scale is something to obsess over. It either makes us feel good or bad each day and yet has no true value. If we're losing weight, our pants fit nicer. If we're gaining, they don't. Why do we need outside validation?

Deep down it's usually because we're always seeking approval of others. Did you know that certain personalities - especially 'people pleasers' are much more likely to deal with weight issues?

So how do you get to a place where you have unconditional love for yourself? It's tricky and takes a lot of self-reflection.

Action step

Here are some questions to ask yourself and journal on:

- ❯ Why does it bother me if other people are judging how I look?

- ❯ Why does it bother me if people are judging how I eat?

- ❯ What is the worst that can happen if they ARE judging me?

- ❯ Have you ever approached someone who you feel judged by and asked if what you think *they're* thinking is correct?

- ❯ How likely is it just a story in your head that you want to be right about it? Ex: I am unhealthy and unattractive - oh look that person gave me side-eye and is definitely thinking "well she's eating fries, no wonder she's overweight!"

Here's the thing. Most people are too self-absorbed and wondering what you're thinking about them to be giving you much thought! And if you disagree with that, maybe the first step is to call in check what you say about others in your head. Are you the one who is the MOST judgemental?

Really, even if someone IS judging you, that's on them. That's their story - their issues. So who cares what they think!

Love you for you. Because you are pretty stinkin' amazing. Aren't we all!!??

XO,

Susannah

Love unplugging

We all catch ourselves in those negative thought patterns and spirals that we know don't serve us and yet...

When in the moment, it's pretty hard to get out of it. I often find myself not even wanting to try!

But here are some great tools when your head is spinning.

1. Unplug.

Seriously. Visualize yourself unplugging a socket. That is you unplugging from your thoughts. Then don't let your mind go there for the next few minutes. You'll soon remember all of the other things you need to do and think about that day that are much more useful.

The key when your thoughts are spinning is to shift.

2. Equally effective is to focus out. Help someone else. Give someone a call and offer support (in any topic). Give without expecting anything in return. Focus on connection with someone else and then you end up feeling so good, you've forgotten all about your negative thoughts.

I swear, it works like a charm every.single.time!

Whenever I think of me, I am limited. Whenever I think of you, I can play bigger.

3. Last strategy that I find really effective is to name any negative voice inside your head.

Hilda is often telling me I'm not good enough, who am I to try, there's way smarter and more successful people out there that people can listen to. *I tell Hilda to take a hike.*

Lucy is always telling me I should go to the gym more often, stop eating so much chocolate and focus more on my appearance. *I tell Lucy "Get the heck outta here!"*

Patricia is always telling me my emails aren't articulate enough, my presentations need more effort and my live videos are boring. *I tell Patricia "You're not welcome here!"*

Action step

Choose one of these strategies and try it out every day for the next week. Then keep going. According to research it takes anywhere from 30 to 66 days to form a new habit!

When in doubt, focus out.

XO, Susannah

Reflecting Back

We're nearing the end of our series. I'd love to wrap things back around to the beginning. To our vision!

What do you get to be for your family when you achieve your goal?

Action step

Journal yourself in 1 year from now standing in your power, feeling fully accomplished. Think of you where you were before you started and where you anticipate being in one year. Date it for today's date of next year.

Here's an example with a comparison to where I was before I started my intermittent fasting journey:

I can't believe how much has changed in one year. I used to eat breakfast as soon as I woke up, always had a snack after a workout regardless of how close to bedtime it was (had to refuel my muscles!) and was eating constantly throughout the day - whether a healthy snack or a meal. When people asked me about intermittent fasting I pretty much scoffed at the thought. I would think: How can anyone go that long without eating! And why!? Plus, I get super hangry if I don't eat every few hours... *Back in "those days" I felt tired all the time, I needed naps in the middle of the day, I ate way more food than anyone around me it seemed, my headaches were awful and didn't see any sign of improving, my weight was at its all-time high and I had lost so much confidence within. I just didn't feel good about myself and I think the lack in energy left me feeling like a pretty bad mother too.*

Now, I look back and feel sorry that I didn't embrace fasting even sooner. I've always eaten really high quality, nutritious foods so there was clearly something else going on. I should have looked for solutions earlier. Now I am medication free, my headaches are cured, my energy is at an all-time high and I chase my kids around just as often as they do me. I feel productive and focused with my work and any hunger feelings I get during a fast subside almost immediately with a nice hot tea. I have no worries of getting 'hangry' because my mood is actually the most stable it's ever been! Plus I've naturally lost 15 pounds over the course of the journey and I've loved every moment. I'm much more in tune with my body's true hunger signals and I finish each day feeling accomplished. Plus, I know I'm also doing this for my long-term health - when I'm in my 80's I will definitely be thanking myself for starting now! I think it truly is possible to live to 100 now. Just like I hoped for when I was a little kid.

Your turn!!

Happy fasting,

Susannah

Love time

How awesome is it the time that we get back in our lives due to fasting!

On my 24-hr fasting days (every Monday and Thursday), I am by far the most productive person on the planet. *At least I always feel that way haha*. I stay completely focused on my tasks and I never need to get up from my desk to prepare food. Instead, I plan my exercise ahead of time to make sure I don't remain TOO focused and never moving.

But overall - having to prep fewer meals and grocery shop even a little less frequently is such a time saver.

I can only imagine the amount of time I save over the course of a month. Or a year. Imagine the amount of time saved when we hit our 80s!

I also feel I get back a lot of family time. That one is mainly due to having more energy and being fully present when we're together.

But it's more than that too. Since I'm focused on enjoying my meals now, I make sure they're nutritious, filling and fulfilling. I am also feeding my family with the same quality foods as I expect for myself.

I've also switched away from thinking of meals as a way to fuel my body but rather focus on how meals are meant to be quality time. We are nourishing our minds more than anything! Nourishing our minds with connection. Truth is, we connect at a deeper level when we share food with others. Especially when those meals are intentional.

Action step

Journal on why you eat? (other than for nourishment, vitamins, minerals etc). What are the most satisfying/fulfilling meals you have - what are the circumstances? Who are you with? How does fasting play into your family dynamic? What is important around meals for you? Do you make sure to always eat your meals with others if connection is important?

Too often, we're eating on the run and not giving much thought into our meals. My belief is that fasting helps us focus on what's important and brings back the joy to eating. Afterall, there is so much freedom in not having any food restrictions!

Fasting = extra time

Susannah

Gratitude

We have hit day 30 of Fasting with Fervor!!

I am so grateful that all of you have taken the time for yourself to go through this journey of reflection together.

At the end of a yoga class I always love when the instructor gets us to bring our hands together and to our hearts and say Namaste. Thank you to yourself, to everyone in this class and to everyone in the whole wide world.

The fasting community is ever growing. We are all interested in seeing each other succeed.

I am so grateful for each of you. You are all doing the work and trying to figure out a system that is best for you. Best for your health, for your family and for your future self.

Here is our last action step of this program.

Action step

Write out 50 things you're grateful for in life. I can virtually guarantee you'll get stuck at a certain point and you might even have to come back to the list a few times. By 50 though, you'll want to keep going!

For those who have kids, this is such a great activity to do at the dinner table or before bed. We come up with 3 things every night. It's an extra powerful activity with kids, I promise. It's amazing what they come up with once they're used to the routine.

I'd love to share with you my top 50 things I'm grateful for but then you wouldn't do the work yourself and would just agree with my points ;)

So my summary is that I am grateful for my health, my family and that I never need to restrict foods or count calories ever again!

I am also grateful to have gotten to a point where I truly love fasting (it was a bumpy road).

Now, I will continue to **Fast with Fervor.**

I hope you continue to love your journey as well.

Happy Fasting,

XO,

Susannah

More Fasting with Fervor with Susannah

To learn how to continue your journey with Susannah,
connect with her at her website:

www.fastwithfacts.com

On Facebook: Fast With Facts - Susannah Fasting Dietitian

On Instagram: @fast.with.facts_rd

The Unbelievable Freedom Habit Guide Series

If you enjoyed this book and would like to continue your
Unbelievable Freedom journey, there are other titles to collect!

Fasting Feasting Freedom: A 33 Day Habit Creation Guide by Kim Smith

Poster Girl Habits: Creating an Intentional Contentment Practice by Kim Smith

A Superhero You: Activate Your Unstoppable Powers by Barbara Anne Cookson

Embracing Next: An Empty Nest Enjoyment Guide by Kim Smith

The Flow Lane: Creating Life One Thought At A Time by Lynn M Robinson

Script A New Life: A Guide to Lasting Change Creation by Tam Veilleux

Spark Your She: Radiance and Resilience in Your Season of Motherhood by Lindsay Harrington

Stop. Drop. Tap! Emotional Freedom Technique for Confidence & Clarity by Tam Veilleux

Fasting is the Foundation. A Real Man's View of Unbelievable Freedom by Ryan Smith

Keep Talking. Communication Habits for Getting Along All Marriage Long by Kayla and J.R. Cox

Information about all of these workbook-style Habit Guides
can be found at www.unbelievablefreedom.com,
along with links to their Amazon listings.

Believe in Unbelievable Freedom

Enjoy Your Life!

Manufactured by Amazon.ca
Bolton, ON